Instant Pot Fast and Easy

Quick-to-Make Recipes for Smart People.

Gilles Murphy

Sommario

Introduction

This full and beneficial guide to instant pot food preparation with over 1000 dishes for breakfast, dinner, dinner, as well as also treats! This is among one of the most extensive immediate pot recipe books ever before released thanks to its variety and also accurate   instructions. Innovative dishes and standards, modern-day take on family members's most enjoyed dishes-- all this is delicious, straightforward as well as certainly as healthy and balanced as it can be. Modification the way you cook with these ingenious immediate pot guidelines. Required a brand-new dinner or a treat? Right here you are! Best instantaneous pot meals collaborated in a few easy steps, also a newbie can do it! The immediate pot specifies the means you prepare everyday. This immediate pot cookbook helps you make the absolute most out of your weekly menu.

The only instant pot publication you will ever before need with the ultimate collection of recipes will assist you in the direction of a simpler and also healthier cooking area experience. If you want to conserve time cooking dishes a lot more successfully, if you intend to provide your family food that can please even the pickiest eater, you are in the ideal location! Master your immediate pot and also make your cooking requires fit into your hectic way of living.

Lunch

Cucumber Salad in Jar

Prep time: 10 minutes

Cooking time: 15 minutes

Servings: 4

Ingredients:

- 1-pound chicken breast, boneless, skinless
- 1 teaspoon ground black pepper
- ½ teaspoon paprika
- ½ teaspoon ground coriander
- 1 tablespoon butter
- 1 cup spinach, chopped
- 1 cucumber, chopped
- 1 teaspoon chili flakes
- 1 teaspoon lemon juice
- 1 teaspoon avocado oil
- 1 cup lettuce, chopped
- 1 cup water for cooking

Directions:

1. Rub the chicken breast with ground black pepper, paprika, and ground coriander.
2. Then place chicken breast in the cooker. Add water.
3. Close the lid and cook the chicken on High-pressure mode for 15 minutes.
4. Make a quick pressure release.
5. Remove chicken breast from the cooker and chill it little. Meanwhile, in the mixing bowl combine together lettuce and spinach.
6. Sprinkle the greens with chili flakes, lemon juice, and avocado oil. Add cucumber and mix up the mixture.
7. Shred the chicken breast and mix it up with butter.
8. Then fill the serving jars with shredded chicken and add green salad mixture. Store the salad in the fridge.

Nutrition: calories 174, fat 6.1, fiber 1, carbs 4, protein 25

Brie Cheese in Pastry

Prep time: 10 minutes

Cooking time: 10 minutes

Servings: 8

Ingredients:

- 10 oz round brie cheese
- 10 sheets phyllo dough
- 1 tablespoon butter
- 1 teaspoon Erythritol

Directions:

1. Place Brie cheese on phyllo pastry and sprinkle it with Erythritol. Add butter and wrap cheese carefully.
2. Place Bre cheese on the trivet of the cooker and lower the air fryer lid.

3. Cook the meal for 10 minutes. Then chill it for 3-5 minutes and cut into the servings.

Nutrition: calories 204, fat 11.1, fiber 0.6, carbs 7, protein 7.4

Pulled Beef

Prep time: 20 minutes

Cooking time: 30 minutes

Servings: 4

Ingredients:

- 12 oz beef, boneless
- 1 cup of water
- ½ cup cream
- 1 teaspoon butter
- 1 teaspoon salt
- 4 oz Parmesan, grated
- 1 teaspoon tomato paste
- 1 teaspoon chili flakes
- 1 teaspoon turmeric
- 1 teaspoon dried cilantro

Directions:

1. Pour water and cream in the cooker. Add beef and salt.

2. Close the lid and cook the meal on High-pressure mode for 30 minutes.

3. Then allow natural pressure release for 10 minutes.

4. Open the lid and shred the meat with the help of the fork.

5. Add butter, tomato paste, chili flakes, turmeric, and dried cilantro. Mix it up.

6. Sprinkle the pulled meat with grated cheese and stir gently. Let the cheese melt.

7. Transfer the cooked pulled beef in the serving bowls.

Nutrition: calories 280, fat 14.1, fiber 0.2, carbs 2.6, protein 35.3

Mushroom and Cheese Sandwich

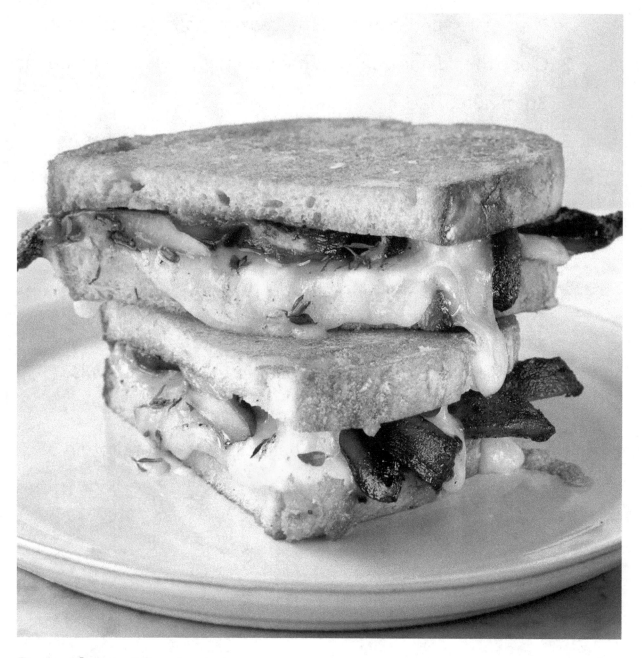

Prep time: 10 minutes

Cooking time: 6 minutes

Servings: 2

Ingredients:

- 2 Portobello mushroom hats

- 3 oz Cheddar cheese, sliced

- 1 tablespoon fresh cilantro, chopped

- ½ teaspoon ground black pepper

- 2 teaspoons butter

- 2 bacon slices

Directions:

1. Remove the flesh from mushrooms. Then sprinkle the vegetables with chopped cilantro and ground black pepper.

2. Fill the mushroom hats with sliced bacon and cheese. Add butter.

3. Place the mushrooms in the Foodi cooker and lower the air fryer lid and cook mushroom hats for 6 minutes.

4. When the meal is cooked, transfer it on the serving plate immediately.

Nutrition: calories 307, fat 24.9, fiber 1.2, carbs 3.9, protein 17.7

16

Beans Pasta Bolognese

Prep time: 10 minutes

Cooking time: 14 minutes

Servings: 6

Ingredients:

- 8 ounces black beans pasta
- 1 teaspoon olive oil
- 2 white onions
- 1 cup ground beef
- 3 tablespoons chives
- 1 teaspoon salt
- 4 cups chicken stock
- ½ cup tomato sauce
- 2 tablespoons soy sauce
- 1 teaspoon turmeric
- 1 teaspoon cilantro
- ½ tablespoon paprika

Directions:

1. Peel the onions and slice it. Place the sliced onions in the pressure cooker.

2. Add ground beef, salt, turmeric, cilantro, and paprika.

3. Stir the mixture well and sauté it for 4 minutes. Stir it gently.

4. Remove the mixture from the pressure cooker and add soy sauce, tomato sauce, and chives. Sauté the mixture for 3 minutes.

5. Add the black bean paste and chicken stock.

6. Add ground beef mixture and close the lid. Cook the dish on the instant mode to "Pressure" for 7 minutes.

7. When the dish is cooked, release the remaining pressure and open the lid. Mix up the dish and transfer it to serving plates.

Nutrition: calories 99, fat 2.1, fiber 5.5, carbs 11.7, protein 10

Lettuce Chicken Salad

Prep time: 15 minutes

Cooking time: 30 minutes

Servings: 6

Ingredients:

- 5 ounces romaine lettuce
- 3 medium tomatoes
- 2 cucumber
- 1 tablespoon olive oil
- 1 teaspoon cayenne pepper
- 1 pound chicken breast
- 1 teaspoon basil
- 1 tablespoon apple cider vinegar
- 1 teaspoon ground black pepper
- 3 ounces black olives
- 1 teaspoon salt
- ½ lemon

Directions:

1. Sprinkle the chicken breast with the basil, salt, apple cider vinegar, and cayenne pepper, and stir it carefully.

2. Transfer the meat to the pressure cooker and close the lid. Set the pressure cooker mode to "Sear/Sauté," and cook for 30 minutes.

3. Meanwhile, chop the lettuce roughly. Slice the olives and chop the cucumbers and tomatoes.

4. Combine the vegetables together in a mixing bowl. Sprinkle the dish with the olive oil. Squeeze the lemon juice.

5. When the chicken is cooked, remove it from the pressure cooker and let the meat rest briefly. Slice the chicken into medium pieces.

6. Add the sliced meat in the mixing bowl. Mix the salad using wooden spoons.

Nutrition: calories 141, fat 8.1, fiber 2, carbs 8.82, protein 9

Spaghetti Bolognese

Prep time: 10 minutes

Cooking time: 10 minutes

Servings: 6

Ingredients:

- 15 ounces spaghetti squash
- 2 cups of water
- 1 cup ground beef
- 1 teaspoon salt
- 1 tablespoon paprika
- 1 teaspoon sour cream
- ⅓ cup tomato paste
- 1 teaspoon thyme

Directions:

1. Combine the ground beef, salt, paprika, sour cream, tomato paste, and thyme together in a mixing bowl. Blend the mixture well until smooth.

2. Place the mixture in the pressure cooker. Set the pressure cooker mode to "Sauté," and cook the mixture for 10 minutes, stirring frequently.

3. Remove the mixture from the pressure cooker. Pour water in the pressure cooker. Cut the spaghetti squash into four parts, and transfer it in the steamer insert.

4. Close the pressure cooker lid and cook the spaghetti squash at the pressure cooker mode for 10 minutes.

5. Let the spaghetti squash rest briefly. Use one or two forks to remove the spaghetti squash strands.

6. Combine the mixture with the ground meat mixture. Mix up the dish and serve it warm.

Nutrition: calories 109, fat 5.5, fiber 2, carbs 7.18, protein 9

Paprika Soup

Prep time: 10 minutes

Cooking time: 45 minutes

Servings: 8

Ingredients:

- 2 white onions
- 1 teaspoon salt
- 2 tablespoons sour cream
- 5 cups chicken stock
- ½ cup cream
- 1 teaspoon paprika
- 2 sweet bell pepper
- 1 pound boneless thighs
- 4 carrots

Directions:

1. Peel the onion and chop it. Peel the carrot and grate it.

2. Place the cream and chicken stock in the pressure cooker. Add thighs and salt.

3. Close the pressure cooker and cook the mixture on the "Sear/Sauté" mode for 25 minutes. Add the sour cream, chopped onion, and carrot.

4. Remove the seeds from the bell peppers and slice them. Add the sliced peppers in the pressure cooker mixture and close the lid.

5. Cook for 20 minutes.

6. When the soup is cooked, remove it from the pressure cooker and sprinkle the dish with the paprika and serve immediately.

Nutrition: calories 111, fat 3.7, fiber 4, carbs 15.98, protein 6

Lunch Cream Soup

Prep time: 10 minutes

Cooking time: 3 hours

Servings: 10

Ingredients:

- 1 pound garlic clove
- 1 teaspoon salt
- 1 cup cream
- ½ cup almond milk
- 5 cups of water
- 1 teaspoon basil
- 1 teaspoon oregano
- ½ teaspoon lemon juice
- 6 oz turnip
- 1 teaspoon ground black pepper
- 1 tablespoon butter

Directions:

1. Peel the garlic cloves and slice them.

2. Combine the cream, almond milk, and water together in a mixing bowl. Add basil, oregano, lemon juice, and ground black pepper.

3. Peel the turnips and chop them.

4. Add the chopped turnips to the cream mixture. Place the cream mixture in the pressure cooker. Add the sliced garlic and butter.

5. Close the pressure cooker lid, and set the mode to "Slow cook". Cook the soup for 3 hours.

6. When all the ingredients of the soup are soft, remove it from the pressure cooker and blend using a blender until smooth.

7. Ladle the soup into the serving bowls.

Nutrition: calories 101, fat 2.9, fiber 1.4, carbs 17.2, protein 3.3

Chicken Salad

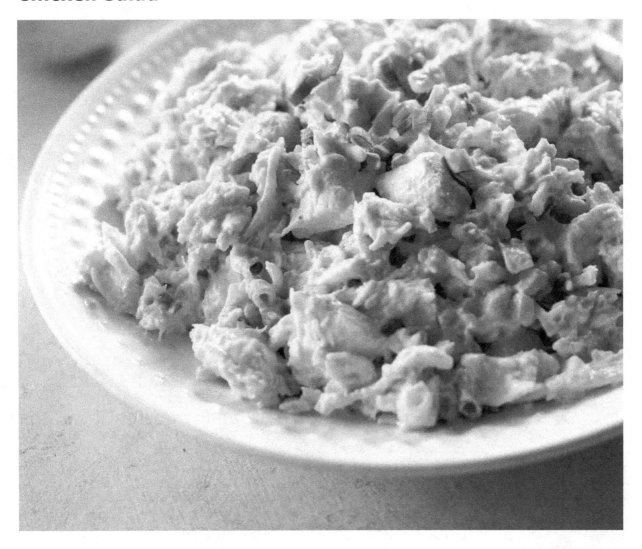

Prep time: 15 minutes

Cooking time: 35 minutes

Servings: 6

Ingredients:

- 1 cup walnuts

- ½ cup cranberries
- 1 pound chicken
- 1 cup plain yogurt
- 1 teaspoon salt
- 1 teaspoon cilantro
- ½ cup fresh dill
- 2 cups of water

Directions:

1. Sprinkle the chicken with salt and transfer it to the pressure cooker.

2. Add water and close the lid. Set the pressure cooker mode to "Sear/Sauté," and cook for 35 minutes.

3. Meanwhile, crush the walnuts and chop the cranberries. Place all the ingredients in a big mixing bowl.

4. Chop the fresh dill and combine it with the yogurt. Stir the mixture well until smooth. Add the cilantro and stir.

5. When the chicken is cooked, remove it from the pressure cooker and shred it. Add the shredded chicken to the salad mixture.

6. Sprinkle the dish with the yogurt mixture. Mix the salad carefully until combined. Serve the salad immediately.

Nutrition: calories 287, fat 15.3 fiber 2.3, carbs 8, protein 30

Spicy Red Soup

Prep time: 15 minutes

Cooking time: 35 minutes

Servings: 6

Ingredients:

- 1 pound tomatoes
- 4 cups beef stock
- 1 teaspoon thyme
- 1 teaspoon coriander
- 1 teaspoon cilantro
- 1 tablespoon ground black pepper
- ½ tablespoon red chili flakes
- 1 teaspoon turmeric
- 2 tablespoons sour cream
- 5 ounces Parmesan cheese
- 1 teaspoon salt
- 1 jalapeno pepper
- 2 yellow onions
- 4 ounces celery stalks

- 1 bay leaf
- ⅓ cup tomato paste

Directions:

1. Wash the tomatoes and remove the skin from the vegetables.
2. Chop the tomatoes. Combine the thyme, coriander, cilantro, ground black pepper, chili flakes, turmeric, and salt together in a mixing bowl.
3. Stir the mixture well. Place the beef stock and chopped tomatoes in the pressure cooker. Add spice mixture.
4. Remove the seeds from the jalapeno pepper and add it to the tomato mixture. Add bay leaf and close the lid.
5. Cook the dish on the "Sauté" mode for 15 minutes. Meanwhile, peel the onions. Chop the onions and celery stalks and add the vegetables to the tomato mixture.
6. Add the sour cream and close the lid. Cook for 20 minutes. Meanwhile, grate the Parmesan cheese.

7. When the soup is cooked, ladle it into the serving bowls. Sprinkle the dish with the grated cheese and serve it immediately.

Nutrition: calories 144, fat 6.6, fiber 3.1, carbs 11.9, protein 11.6

Cheddar Soup

Prep time: 15 minutes

Cooking time: 40 minutes

Servings: 8

Ingredients:

- 8 ounces broccoli
- ½ cup parsley
- 10 ounces beef brisket
- 1 teaspoon salt
- 1 tablespoon sour cream
- 7 cups of water
- 1 carrot
- 1 cup green beans
- 10 ounces cheddar cheese
- 1 teaspoon cilantro
- 1 teaspoon ground black pepper
- ¼ cup coriander leaves
- 1 teaspoon lemon juice

Directions:

1. Place the broccoli, beef brisket, green beans, and salt in the pressure cooker.

2. Peel the carrot and chop it. Add the chopped carrot and water in the pressure cooker too. Close the lid and cook the dish on the "Pressure Cooker" mode for 30 minutes.

3. Remove the pressure cooker vessel from the pressure cooker machine carefully. Discard the beef brisket and set aside. Blend the mixture until smooth.

4. Place the pressure cooker vessel into the pressure cooker machine again.

5. Add sour cream, cilantro, ground black pepper, and lemon juice. Chop the parsley and coriander leaves and add them to the soup.

6. Grate the cheddar cheese.

7. Sprinkle the mixture with the cheese and cook the soup for 10 minutes. When the cooking time ends, the cheese should be melted.

8. Mix the soup carefully until you get a smooth texture. Remove the soup from the pressure cooker and add beef brisket.

9. Ladle the soup into the serving bowls and serve.

Nutrition: calories 152, fat 8.9, fiber 2, carbs 7.15, protein 11

Oregano Rolls

Prep time: 10 minutes

Cooking time: 25 minutes

Servings: 8

Ingredients:

- 1 cup cauliflower rice, cooked
- 1 tablespoon curry
- 1 teaspoon salt
- ½ teaspoon tomato paste
- ¼ cup cream
- 1 cup chicken stock
- 1 teaspoon oregano
- 1 pound kale
- 1 teaspoon olive oil
- 1 yellow onion
- 3 tablespoons chives
- 1 tablespoon paprika
- ½ tablespoon ground black pepper

- 1 teaspoon garlic powder
- 1 egg
- 1 cup beef stock

Directions:

1. Combine the cooked cauliflower rice and curry together in a mixing bowl.
2. Beat the egg in the mixture. Peel the yellow onion and chop it.
3. Chop the chives and add the vegetables to a mixing bowl too. Sprinkle the dish with the salt, oregano, paprika, ground black pepper, and garlic powder.
4. Blend the mixture well using your hands until smooth.
5. Separate the kale into leaves.
6. Put the cauliflower rice mixture in the middle of every kale leave and roll them.
7. Combine the tomato paste, cream, chicken stock, olive oil, and beef stock together and stir the mixture. Transfer the kale rolls in the pressure cooker.

8. Add tomato paste mixture and close the lid. Set the pressure cooker mode to "Sauté," and cook for 25 minutes.

9. When the cooking time ends, open the lid and let the dish rest briefly.

10. Transfer the kale rolls in the serving plates, sprinkle it with the tomato sauce, and serve.

Nutrition: calories 66, fat 2, fiber 2.3, carbs 9.9, protein 3.7

Coconut Spinach Casserole

Prep time: 15 minutes

Cooking time: 25 minutes

Servings: 6

Ingredients:

- 2 cups spinach
- 1 cup cream
- 3 tablespoons coconut flour
- 1 teaspoon salt
- 8 ounces Parmesan cheese
- 2 onions
- 1 teaspoon oregano
- ½ teaspoon red chili flakes
- 1 cup green peas

Directions:

1. Wash the spinach and chop it well. Transfer the chopped spinach into a mixing bowl.

2. Peel the onions and dice them.

3. Combine the salt, coconut flour, and chili flakes together in the separate bowl. Add oregano and cream. Whisk the mixture until smooth.

4. Grate the Parmesan cheese. Place the peas in the pressure cooker and sprinkle it with a small amount of the grated cheese to create the thin layer.

5. Add the diced onion and sprinkle the dish with the cheese again. Add the chopped spinach and add all remaining cheese.

6. Pour the cream mixture and close the lid.

7. Set the pressure cooker mode to "Steam," and cook for 25 minutes.

8. When the cooking time ends, let it rest. Transfer the dish to a serving plate.

Nutrition: calories 200, fat 11, fiber 3.6, carbs 12, protein 15

Stuffed Meatloaf

Prep time: 15 minutes

Cooking time: 30 minutes

Servings: 8

Ingredients:

- 2 cups ground beef
- 3 eggs, boiled, peeled
- 1 tablespoon flax meal
- 1 teaspoon salt
- 1 teaspoon chili flakes
- 1 teaspoon ground coriander
- 1 tablespoon butter
- 1 cup water, for cooking

Directions:

1. Place ground beef in the mixing bowl. Add flax meal and salt.

2. After this, add chili flakes and ground coriander. Mix up the ground beef mixture very carefully.

3. Pour water in Foodi Pressure cooker and insert trivet.

4. Take the loaf mold and spread it with butter generously. Place the ground beef mixture into the loaf mold and flatten well.

5. Place the boiled eggs inside the ground beef mixture.

6. Flatten the ground beef mixture again to cover the eggs totally. Cover the mold with the foil and secure the edges.

7. Place it on the trivet and close the lid.

8. Cook the meal on the High-pressure mode for 30 minutes.

9. Then allow natural pressure release for 10 minutes. Chill the meatloaf well and then slice it.

Nutrition: calories 105, fat 7.5, fiber 0.3, carbs 0.4, protein 8.8

Lunch Schnitzel

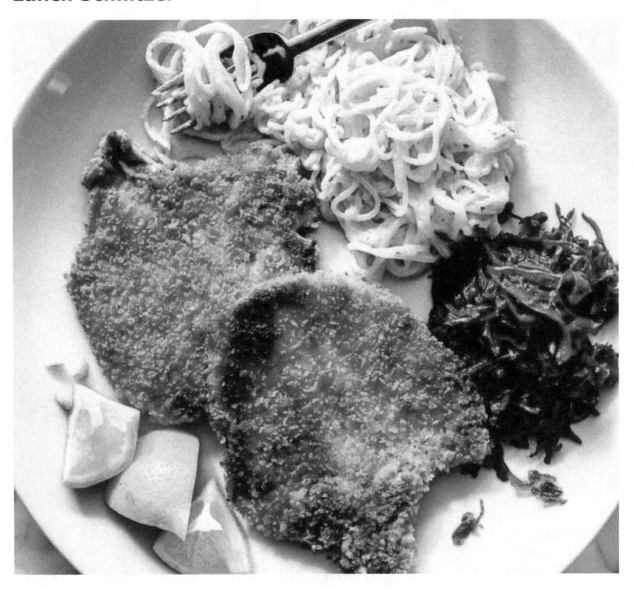

Prep time: 10 minutes

Cooking time: 16 minutes

Servings: 6

Ingredients:

- 1 pound pork chops

- 1 teaspoon salt

- 1 teaspoon turmeric

- 2 eggs

- ¼ cup of coconut milk

- 1 teaspoon cilantro

- ½ cup coconut flour

- 1 teaspoon lemon juice

- 1 teaspoon ground black pepper

Directions:

1. Beat the pork chops carefully. Combine the salt, turmeric, cilantro, and ground black pepper together and stir the mixture.

2. Rub the pork chops with the spice mixture. Sprinkle the meat with the lemon juice and leave it for 10 minutes to marinate.

3. Meanwhile, beat the eggs in a mixing bowl. Blend them with a whisk, then add the milk and stir. Dip the pork chops in the egg mixture.

4. Dip the pork chops in the flour. Add a splash of olive oil to the pressure cooker and preheat it using "Sauté."

5. Transfer the coated pork chops to the pressure cooker.

6. Cook the schnitzels for 8 minutes from each side. Let the meat rest and serve.

Nutrition: calories 258, fat 25.2, fiber 6.4, carbs 10.2, protein 22.2

Stuffed Mozzarella Caprese

Prep time: 15 minutes

Cooking time: 30 minutes

Servings: 6

Ingredients:

- 13 oz chicken breast, skinless, boneless
- 1 tomato, sliced
- ½ cup fresh basil
- 5 oz Mozzarella, sliced
- ½ teaspoon salt
- 1 tablespoon butter
- 1 teaspoon paprika
- 1 tablespoon olive oil
- 1 teaspoon chili flakes
- ½ teaspoon turmeric
- 1 cup water, for cooking

Directions:

1. Beat the chicken breast gently with the help of the smooth side of the kitchen hammer. Then make a longitudinal cut in the breast (to get the pocket).

2. Chop the fresh basil roughly. Rub the chicken breast with salt, paprika, chili flakes, and turmeric.

3. Then fill it with sliced Mozzarella, butter, and chopped fresh basil. Brush the chicken breast with olive oil and wrap into the foil.

4. Pour water in the Foodi cooker and insert trivet.

5. Transfer the chicken breast on the trivet and close the lid. Cook the meal on High-pressure mode for 30 minutes.

6. After this, use quick pressure release and discard foil from the chicken. Slice it and transfer on the serving plates.

Nutrition: calories 182, fat 11.2, fiber 0.3, carbs 1.3, protein 18.5

Veggie and Beef Lasagna

Prep time: 15 minutes

Cooking time: 35 minutes

Servings: 6

Ingredients:

- 1 cup ground beef
- 1 cup tomato juice
- 9 ounces zucchini, sliced
- 1 tablespoon butter
- 1 teaspoon sour cream
- ½ cup half and half
- 10 ounces Parmesan cheese
- ½ cup cream cheese
- 1 white onion
- 1 teaspoon ground black pepper
- 1 teaspoon cilantro
- ½ teaspoon salt
- ½ cup beef stock

Directions:

1. Combine the tomato juice, sour cream, half and half, beef stock and salt together in a mixing bowl. Stir the mixture well.

2. Grate the Parmesan cheese and peel and slice the onion. Combine the ground beef with the ground black pepper and cilantro and stir the mixture.

3. Then add the butter in the pressure cooker and the ground beef mixture and cook it on "Sauté" mode until it is cooked (approximately 10 minutes), stirring frequently.

4. Remove the ground beef from the pressure cooker. Place the sliced zucchini in the pressure cooker and pour the tomato juice mixture to cover the zucchini.

5. Add the layer of the sliced onion, grated cheese, and ground beef mixture. Continue to make the layers until you use all the ingredients.

6. Close the lid, and set the manual mode for 25 minutes. When the dish is cooked, let it cool briefly and serve.

Nutrition: calories 330, fat 24.1, fiber 1.1, carbs 8.2, protein 22.9

Meat Taco

Prep time: 10 minutes

Cooking time: 35 minutes

Servings: 6

Ingredients:

- 1 pound ground pork
- ½ cup spinach
- ½ cup cilantro
- 1 tablespoon salt
- 1 teaspoon oregano
- 1 teaspoon cumin
- ½ teaspoon ground coriander
- 1 teaspoon ground black pepper
- 1 teaspoon cayenne pepper
- 1 tablespoon onion powder
- 2 cups chicken stock
- 1 tablespoon tomato paste
- 1 tablespoon olive oil

Directions:

1. Wash the spinach and cilantro and chop them. Transfer the mixture to a mixing bowl.

2. Add ground pork and sprinkle the mixture with the salt, oregano, and cumin.

3. Blend the mixture. Transfer the mixture to the pressure cooker and sprinkle it with the olive oil.

4. Sauté it for 10 minutes, stirring frequently.

5. Add the ground black pepper, onion powder, and tomato paste. Add chicken stock and blend well.

6. Cook the taco meat at the pressure cooker mode to "Pressure," and cook for 25 minutes.

7. When the taco meat is cooked, let it rest briefly and serve it with tortillas.

Nutrition: calories 286, fat 19.1, fiber 1, carbs 5.53, protein 22

Fresh Cottage Cheese

Prep time: 5 minutes

Cooking time: 5 minutes

Servings: 5

Ingredients:

- 6 cups almond milk
- ¼ cup apple cider vinegar
- 1 teaspoon salt
- ⅓ cup sour cream
- 3 tablespoons Erythritol
- ⅓ cup almonds

Directions:

1. Place the almond milk in the pressure cooker and close the lid.

2. Set the pressure cooker mode to "Slow cook", and cook the almond milk with the lid open until it becomes to boil.

3. Whisk the almond milk frequently and add salt. Add the vinegar gradually.

4. Close the lid and unplug the pressure cooker. Leave the almond milk for 25 minutes. Cover the sieve with the cheesecloth and strain the cheese into it.

5. Squeeze it well to get rid of the whey.

6. Transfer the cheese into a blender and blend it well.

7. Add Erythritol and sour cream. Blend the mixture for 3 minutes.

8. Transfer the cottage cheese into the serving bowls and sprinkle it with the almonds and serve.

Nutrition: calories 120, fat 10, fiber 0.8, carbs 2.1, protein 3

Lunch Tortillas

Prep time: 10 minutes

Cooking time: 8 minutes

Servings: 5

Ingredients:

- 5 almond flour tortillas
- 8 ounces ham
- ½ cup lettuce
- ¼ cup tomato paste
- 6 ounces tomatoes
- 1 red onion
- 1 teaspoon salt
- 1 teaspoon ground black pepper
- 1 teaspoon oregano
- 3 tablespoons lemon juice

Directions:

1. Chop the ham and lettuce. Slice the tomatoes and onions.

2. Combine the salt, ground black pepper, and oregano together and stir the mixture. Spread the tortillas with the tomato paste.

3. Sprinkle the tortillas with the lettuce, ham, sliced onions, and tomatoes.

4. Add the spice mixture and lemon juice. Wrap the tortillas and place them in the pressure cooker. Set the manual mode at 8 minutes.

5. When the cooking time ends, remove the wraps from the pressure cooker and serve the dish hot.

Nutrition: calories 195, fat 9, fiber 4.7, carbs 13.2, protein 6

Mushroom and Cream Bowl

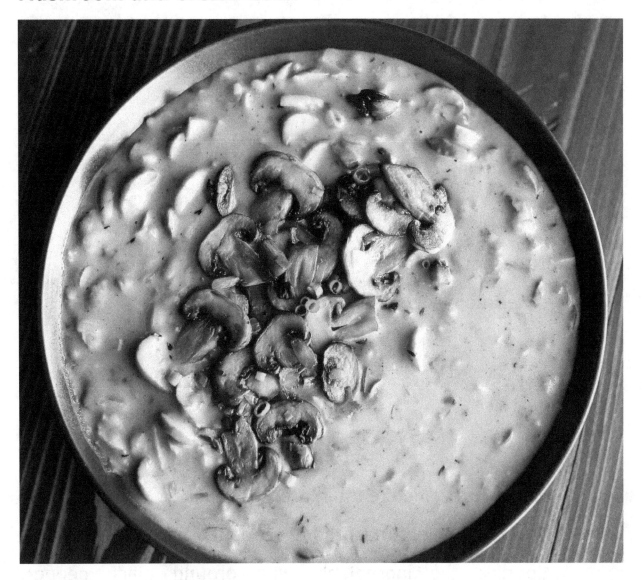

Prep time: 10 minutes

Cooking time: 2 hours

Servings: 3

Ingredients:

- 1 ½ cup white mushrooms, chopped
- 5 oz bacon, chopped
- 2 tablespoons butter
- 1 white onion, diced
- 1 teaspoon salt
- 1 teaspoon ground black pepper
- ½ cup cream
- 1 teaspoon oregano
- ¾ teaspoon cayenne pepper

Directions:

1. Place butter and cream in pressure cooker.

2. Add diced onion, mushrooms, chopped bacon, and salt.

3. Sprinkle the ingredients with ground black pepper, oregano, and cayenne pepper. Mix up well.

4. Close the lid and cook the meal on Low-pressure mode for 2 hours.

5. When the time is over, open the lid and stir the cooked meal with the spoon well.

6. Transfer it into the serving bowls and serve warm.

Nutrition: calories 376, fat 29.9, fiber 1.7, carbs 7.5, protein 19.6

Keto Pizza

Prep time: 15 minutes

Cooking time: 35 minutes

Servings: 12

Ingredients:

- 8 ounces soda keto dough
- 1 egg
- ½ cup tomatoes
- 6 ounces pepperoni
- 5 ounces mozzarella cheese
- 3 tablespoons tomato paste
- 1 tablespoon sour cream
- 1 teaspoon oregano
- 2 tablespoons basil
- 4 ounces black olives
- 1 tablespoon fresh cilantro
- 1 teaspoon olive oil

Directions:

1. Roll the dough using a rolling pin in the shape of the circle.

2. Spray the pressure cooker inside with olive oil and line with the pizza crust.

3. Combine the tomato paste and sour cream together and stir the mixture. Spread the pizza crust with the tomato mixture.

4. Slice the pepperoni and black olives. Sprinkle the pizza crust with the sliced ingredients. Grate the cheddar cheese.

5. Chop the cilantro and sprinkle the pizza with it.

6. Slice the tomatoes and add them to the pizza crust. Add grated cheese, basil, and oregano.

7. Sprinkle the pizza with the grated cheese and close the lid. Cook the dish on the manual mode for 35 minutes.

8. When the cooking time ends, open the lid and let the pizza rest. Transfer it to serving plates and slice it into serving pieces.

Nutrition: calories 187, fat 11.5, fiber 1, carbs 12.2, protein 8.7

Calzone

Prep time: 10 minutes

Cooking time: 35 minutes

Servings: 7

Ingredients:

- 6 ounces soda dough
- 1 cup ricotta cheese
- 8 ounces ham
- 7 ounces Parmesan cheese
- 1 tablespoon butter
- 1 teaspoon paprika
- 1 teaspoon lemon juice

Directions:

1. Roll the soda dough using a rolling pin.
2. Grate the Parmesan cheese and chop the ham.

3. Sprinkle the one part of the rolled dough with the grated cheese and chopped ham. Add the ricotta cheese.

4. Sprinkle the mixture with the paprika and wrap it to make the calzone. Add the butter in the pressure cooker and melt it.

5. Transfer the calzone to the machine and sprinkle it with the lemon juice. Close the lid, and set the manual for 35 minutes.

6. You can turn the calzone into another side once during the cooking.

7. When the dish is cooked, remove it from the pressure cooker and serve.

Nutrition: calories 249, fat 14.2, fiber 0.8, carbs 11.4, protein 19.6

Black Pasta Salad

Prep time: 10 minutes

Cooking time: 20 minutes

Servings: 6

Ingredients:

- 5 ounces black bean pasta
- ½ lemon
- 3 cups chicken stock
- 2 tomatoes
- ½ cup pork rind
- 3 tablespoons mayonnaise
- ½ cup lettuce
- 1 teaspoon basil
- 1 teaspoon paprika
- 5 ounces Romano cheese
- ½ cup cream
- 5 ounces sliced bacon, fried

Directions:

1. Place the pasta and chicken stock in the pressure cooker.

2. Add paprika and basil and stir the mixture.

3. Close the pressure cooker and set the mode to "Pressure." Cook for 20 minutes. Meanwhile, tear the lettuce and place it in the mixing bowl.

4. Squeeze the lemon juice from the lemon and sprinkle the lettuce with the juice. Combine the mayonnaise and cream together.

5. Stir the mixture well. Chop the Romano cheese and fried bacon. Slice the tomatoes and cut each slice in half.

6. When the pasta is cooked, remove it from the pressure cooker and rinse it with hot water. Add the pasta to the lettuce mixture.

7. Add sliced tomatoes, Romano cheese, and fried bacon.

8. Sprinkle the dish with the cream sauce and pork rinds.

9. Blend the mixture well. Transfer it to serving plates.

Nutrition: calories 392, fat 23.6, fiber 5.9, carbs 13.5, protein 32.4

California Sandwich

Prep time: 10 minutes

Cooking time: 4 minutes

Servings: 6

Ingredients:

- 5 ounces keto naan bread
- 1 teaspoon sesame seeds
- 1 tablespoon mustard
- 2 tablespoons lemon juice
- 3 tablespoons garlic sauce
- 5 ounces cheddar cheese
- ¼ cup sunflower sprouts
- 1 teaspoon onion powder
- 1 avocado, pitted
- 8 ounces smoked chicken
- 1 teaspoon butter

Directions:

1. Combine the mustard, lemon juice, garlic sauce, and onion powder together.

2. Stir the mixture well. Spread all the keto naan bread slices with the mustard sauce.

3. Slice cheddar cheese. Slice the avocado.

4. Chop the smoked chicken. Place the sliced cheese, avocado, and chopped smoked chicken into 3 bread slices.

5. Sprinkle it with the sesame seeds. Cover the mixture with the naan bread slices to make the sandwiches.

6. Add the butter in the pressure cooker. Transfer the sandwiches in the pressure cooker and set the mode to "Sauté."

7. Cook the sandwiches for 2 minutes on each side.

8. Transfer the cooked dish in the serving plates. Cut them in half and serve.

Nutrition: calories 264, fat 17.2, fiber 2.8, carbs 8.7, protein 18.8

Miso Soup

Prep time: 8 minutes

Cooking time: 10 minutes

Servings: 6

Ingredients:

- 1 tablespoon miso paste
- 1 teaspoon turmeric
- ½ tablespoon ground ginger
- 1 teaspoon cilantro
- 5 cups chicken stock
- 5 ounces celery stalk
- 1 teaspoon salt
- 1 tablespoon sesame seeds
- 1 teaspoon lemon zest
- ½ cup of soy sauce
- 1 white onion

Directions:

1. Combine the turmeric, ground ginger, cilantro, salt, lemon zest, and chicken stock together in the pressure cooker.

2. Peel the onion. Chop the celery stalk and white onion.

3. Add the vegetables in the pressure cooker.

4. Blend the mixture and close the lid. Set the pressure cooker mode to "Pressure," and cook for 8 minutes.

5. Add the miso paste and soy sauce.

6. Stir the mixture well until the miso paste dissolves. Cook for 2 minutes.

7. Ladle the soup into serving bowls.

Nutrition: calories 155, fat 7.3, fiber 1, carbs 14.66, protein 7

Chicken Burrito

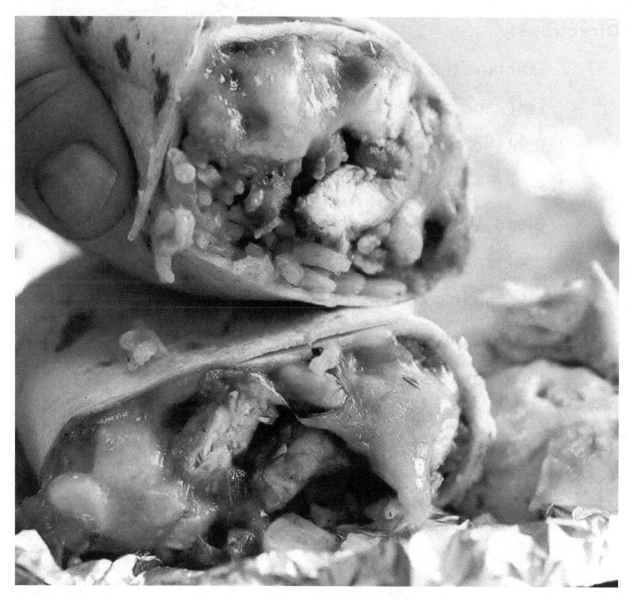

Prep time: 10 minutes

Cooking time: 35 minutes

Servings: 5

Ingredients:

- 3 tablespoons chipotle paste

- 1 pound chicken

- 2 cups of water

- 1 tablespoon tomato paste

- 1 teaspoon cayenne pepper

- 5 keto tortillas

- 1 teaspoon mayo sauce

- 1 tablespoon garlic powder

- ⅓ cup fresh parsley

- 3 ounces lettuce

- ¼ cup of salsa

Directions:

1. Chop the chicken roughly and place it in the pressure cooker. Add cayenne pepper, garlic powder, and chili pepper.

2. Pour water and close the lid. Set the pressure cooker mode to "Sear/Sauté," and cook the meat for 30 minutes.

3. Meanwhile, tear the lettuce into a mixing bowl.

4. Add salsa and mayo sauce. Blend the mixture well. Spread the keto tortillas with the salsa and chipotle paste.

5. Chop the parsley, and separate it evenly between all tortillas. Add tomato paste and lettuce mixture.

6. When the chicken is cooked, shred it well and transfer the meat in the tortillas. Wrap the tortillas to make the burritos.

7. Transfer the burritos in the pressure cooker and cook the dish on the "Sauté" mode for 5 minutes.

8. When the cooking time ends, remove the dish from the pressure cooker. Serve it immediately.

Nutrition: calories 244, fat 7.6, fiber 2.5, carbs 10.4, protein 32.6

Lettuce and Tuna Salad

Prep time: 15 minutes

Cooking time: 20 minutes

Servings: 6

Ingredients:

- 1 pound fresh tuna
- 2 red onions
- 2 bell peppers
- 1 cup lettuce
- ⅓ cup pecans
- 2 tablespoons lemon juice
- 1 teaspoon olive oil
- 2 tablespoons butter
- ½ teaspoon rosemary
- ¼ cup cream
- 5 ounces tomatoes
- 1 teaspoon salt
- ½ cup of water

Directions:

1. Sprinkle the tuna with the rosemary and salt and stir it gently.

2. Tadd the butter in the pressure cooker and add the tuna.

3. Add water and close the lid. Set the pressure cooker mode to "Pressure," and cook the fish for 20 minutes.

4. Meanwhile, peel the onions and slice them.

5. Chop the lettuce and bell peppers.

6. Chop the tomatoes and crush the pecans.

7. Place the lemon juice, olive oil, and cream in the mixing bowl and stir the mixture well. Place all the vegetables in the mixing bowl and stir the mixture gently.

8. When the tuna is cooked, remove it from the pressure cooker and shred it.

9. Add the shredded tuna in the vegetable mixture.

10. Mix up the salad using two spoons.

11. Transfer the salad in the serving bowl and sprinkle it with the cream sauce and serve it.

Nutrition: calories 190, fat 11.3, fiber 2, carbs 7.29, protein 17

Carrots Casserole

Prep time: 10 minutes

Cooking time: 40 minutes

Servings: 6

Ingredients:

- 1 pound cabbage
- 2 carrots
- 1 onion
- ½ cup tomato juice
- 5 eggs
- 1 teaspoon salt
- 1 teaspoon paprika
- ½ tablespoon coconut flour
- 1 teaspoon cilantro
- 1 tablespoon butter
- ½ cup pork rinds

Directions:

1. Chop the cabbage and sprinkle it with the salt.

2. Stir the mixture and leave it until the cabbage gives off liquid. Combine the tomato juice with the cilantro.

3. Add the butter in the pressure cooker and melt it.

4. Add the chopped cabbage and sauté it for 10 minutes, stirring frequently. Beat the eggs in the mixing bowl and whisk well.

5. Add flour and stir it until you get a smooth mixture. Add the tomato mixture in the pressure cooker and stir it well.

6. Add egg mixture and pork rinds.

7. Sprinkle the dish with the paprika.

8. Peel the onion and carrots and chop them.

9. Add the chopped ingredients in the pressure cooker and stir the mixture. Close the lid, and set the manual mode for 35 minutes.

10. When the dish is cooked, let it rest briefly and serve.

Nutrition: calories 178, fat 10, fiber 3.2, carbs 9.8, protein 13.8

Home Lunch Baguette

Prep time: 15 minutes

Cooking time: 30 minutes

Servings: 6

Ingredients:

- 2 cups almond flour
- ⅓ cup whey
- 1 teaspoon baking powder
- 1 tablespoon Erythritol
- 1 teaspoon salt
- 5 ounces Parmesan cheese
- 8 ounces Mozzarella cheese
- 1 teaspoon parsley
- 1 teaspoon cilantro
- 1 teaspoon oregano
- 1 tablespoon rosemary
- 2 eggs
- 1 tablespoon butter

- 1 cup fresh spinach

Directions:

1. Combine the whey with the baking powder and stir the mixture well.

2. Add Erythritol, salt, and cilantro and stir the mixture. Add the almond flour and knead the smooth dough.

3. Chop the parsley and combine it with the oregano. Add rosemary, eggs, and butter.

4. Chop the spinach and add it to the parsley mixture.

5. Chop the Mozzarella cheese and grate the Parmesan cheese. Combine the cheese with the green mixture and stir.

6. Fill the dough with spinach mixture and make the form of the baguette. Transfer the dish to the pressure cooker and leave it for 10 minutes.

7. Close the lid, and set the pressure cooker mode to "Pressure." Cook for 30 minutes. Turn it into another side after 15 minutes of cooking.

8. When the baguette is cooked, let it rest briefly and then remove it from the pressure cooker. Slice it and serve warm.

Nutrition: calories 285, fat 20, fiber 1.5, carbs 5.6, protein 23.6

Italian Tart

Prep time: 10 minutes

Cooking time: 25 minutes

Servings: 10

Ingredients:

- 9 ounces sundried tomatoes
- 1 teaspoon salt
- 7 ounces soda dough (keto dough)
- 1 egg yolk
- ¼ cup almond milk
- 2 tablespoons butter
- 2 white onions
- ½ cup pork rinds
- 1 teaspoon nutmeg

Directions:

1. Roll out the soda dough using a rolling pin, and transfer it to the pressure cooker.
2. Put the tomatoes in the rolled dough.
3. Peel the onions and slice them. Add the sliced onion to the tart. Sprinkle the tart with the salt.
4. Add almond milk, butter, and nutmeg. Add the pork rinds. Whisk the egg yolk and sprinkle the tart with the mixture.
5. Close the pressure cooker lid and cook for 25 minutes.
6. When the cooking time ends, release the remaining pressure and remove the tart from the pressure cooker carefully. Cut it into pieces and serve.

Nutrition: calories 218, fat 7.9, fiber 6.4, carbs 21.2, protein 19.4

Warm Lunch Tortillas

Prep time: 15 minutes

Cooking time: 10 minutes

Servings: 6

Ingredients:

- 4 eggs
- 1 teaspoon salt
- ½ teaspoon ground black pepper
- 1 tablespoon olive oil
- 6 keto tortillas
- 4 tablespoons salsa
- 1 teaspoon cilantro
- ½ teaspoon paprika
- 7 ounces beetroot
- 1 teaspoon lemon zest
- 1 medium carrot
- 1 red onion
- 1 tablespoon lemon juice

- 1 cup lettuce

Directions:

1. Beat the eggs in the mixing bowl and whisk them well.

2. Add ground black pepper, salt, cilantro, and paprika. Stir the mixture well.

3. Spray the pressure cooker inside and transfer the egg mixture. Set the pressure cooker mode to "Sauté" and ladle the egg mixture to make the crepe.

4. Cook it on each side for 1 minute. Continue this step with five additional crepes. Chill the crepes.

5. Spread the keto tortillas with the salsa. Sprinkle them with the lemon juice and add lettuce. Add the egg crepes. Cut the carrot into the strips.

6. Chop the beetroot and slice the onion.

7. Add the vegetables into the tortillas.

8. Add lemon zest and make the wraps. Transfer the wraps into the pressure cooker and cook them at the manual mode for 3 minutes.

9. Remove the dish from the pressure cooker and serve hot.

Nutrition: calories 144, fat 8.1, fiber 3, carbs 10.2, protein 8.8

Quick Pie

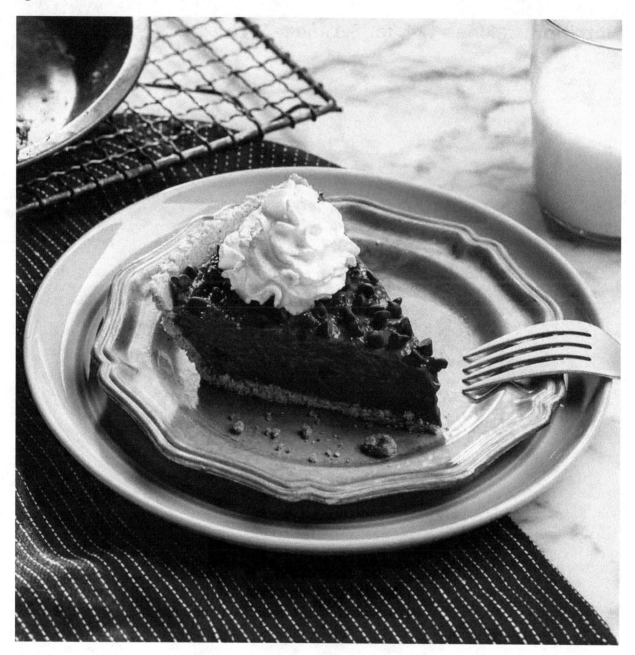

Prep time: 15 minutes

Cooking time: 25 minutes

Servings: 8

Ingredients:

- 2 cups almond flour
- 7 ounces butter
- 1 teaspoon salt
- 1 egg
- ¼ cup almond milk
- 1 pound sausage
- 1 teaspoon tomato paste
- 5 ounces Parmesan cheese
- 1 teaspoon cilantro
- 1 teaspoon oregano
- 3 tablespoons sour cream
- 1 teaspoon turmeric
- 1 carrot

Directions:

1. Combine the butter with the almond flour. Add salt, almond milk, and egg.

2. Knead the dough. Chop the sausages and combine them with the tomato paste.

3. Add the cilantro, oregano, and sour cream. Sprinkle the sausage mixture with the turmeric.

4. Peel the carrot and slice it. Roll the dough into the round form and transfer it into the pressure cooker.

5. Put the sausage mixture in the middle of the dough and flatten it well. Add the sliced carrot and milk.

6. Close the lid, and set the pressure cooker mode to "Pressure." Follow the directions of the pressure cooker. Cook for 25 minutes.

7. Check if the dish is cooked using a wooden spoon and remove it from the pressure cooker. Slice it and serve.

Nutrition: calories 615, fat 56.4, fiber 3.3, carbs 7.6, protein 23

Filo Snail

Prep time: 15 minutes

Cooking time: 30 minutes

Servings: 6

Ingredients:

- 5 sheets filo pastry
- 1 tablespoon sesame seeds
- 1 tablespoon olive oil
- 1 teaspoon butter
- 1 cup spinach
- 1 teaspoon oregano
- ½ teaspoon nutmeg
- 1 teaspoon cilantro
- 1 cup cottage cheese
- 1 teaspoon garlic powder
- 1 egg yolk

Directions:

1. Sprinkle the filo pastry sheets with the olive oil.

2. Chop the spinach and combine it with the oregano, nutmeg, cilantro, cottage cheese, and garlic powder. Stir the mixture well.

3. Place the spinach mixture into the filo pastry sheets and roll them into the shape of the snail. Whisk the egg yolk and sprinkle the "snail" with it.

4. Add sesame seeds and transfer the dish to the pressure cooker.

5. Close the lid, and set the pressure cooker mode to "Pressure."

6. Cook for 30 minutes or until it is cooked.

7. Remove the "snail" from the pressure cooker and rest briefly. Cut it into pieces and serve.

Nutrition: calories 80, fat 5.5, fiber 0, carbs 4.37, protein 4

Puff Rolls

Prep time: 10 minutes

Cooking time: 25 minutes

Servings: 6

Ingredients:

- 7 ounces puff pastry
- 1 teaspoon olive oil
- 1 cup ground beef
- 1 yellow onion
- 1 teaspoon cilantro
- 1 tablespoon cumin
- 1 egg yolk
- 2 tablespoons water
- 1 teaspoon oregano
- ½ teaspoon turmeric
- ½ teaspoon ginger
- 1 teaspoon salt
- ½ tablespoon lemon juice

Directions:

1. Peel the onion and dice it. Combine the diced onion with the cilantro, oregano, turmeric, ginger, and salt.

2. Stir the mixture well and add ground beef. Mix it up.

3. Roll the puff pastry using a rolling pin.

4. Separate it into the medium logs.

5. Add the onion mixture in the puff pastry logs and make long rolls. Whisk the egg yolk with water until blended and add cumin.

6. Sprinkle the pressure cooker with the olive oil inside and transfer the Turkey rolls in the pressure cooker.

7. Brush the logs with the egg mixture.

8. Close the lid, and set the pressure cooker mode to "Pressure," and cook for 25 minutes or until it is done.

9. Remove it from the pressure cooker and rest briefly and serve.

Nutrition: calories 268, fat 18.2, fiber 1, carbs 17.58, protein 9

Garlic Spaghetti

Prep time: 10 minutes

Cooking time: 16 minutes

Servings: 7

Ingredients:

- 6 garlic cloves
- 1 tablespoon garlic powder
- 1 teaspoon onion powder
- 1 tablespoon heavy cream
- 3 tablespoons butter
- 6 ounces Parmesan cheese
- 2 cups chicken stock
- 9 ounces black beans noodles
- ½ cup fresh parsley
- 1 teaspoon white wine
- ½ lemon
- 4 ounces tomatoes
- 1 cup ground chicken

Directions:

1. Cook the black beans noodles to al dente according to the directions on the package. Slice the garlic cloves and combine it with the ground chicken.
2. Add onion powder, garlic powder, cream, white wine, and chicken stock. Blend the mixture.
3. Transfer the mixture to the pressure cooker and sauté it for 6 minutes or until the mixture is cooked.
4. Add the black beans noodles.
5. Chop the tomatoes and add them in the pressure cooker.
6. Grate the Parmesan cheese. Blend the pressure cooker mixture well to not damage the noodles and close the lid.
7. Cook the dish on the pressure mode for 10 minutes. Transfer the cooked dish into the serving plates.
8. Sprinkle it with the grated cheese and serve hot.

Nutrition: calories 302, fat 14, fiber 8.5, carbs 15.5, protein 30.9

Salmon Pie

Prep time: 15 minutes

Cooking time: 35 minutes

Servings: 6

Ingredients:

- 1 pound salmon fillet, boiled
- 1 teaspoon salt
- 7 ounces butter
- 1 cup almond flour
- ½ cup dill
- 1 teaspoon paprika
- 2 tablespoons lemon juice
- 1 teaspoon cilantro
- 5 ounces dried tomatoes
- ¼ cup garlic
- 2 sweet bell peppers
- 1 tablespoon olive oil

Directions:

1. Shred the boiled salmon fillet and sprinkle it with the salt and lemon juice and stir the mixture. Combine the butter with the flour, paprika, and cilantro.

2. Knead the dough. Chop the dill and slice the garlic.

3. Chop the tomatoes and bell peppers. Combine the vegetables together and add the mixture in the shredded salmon.

4. Roll the soft dough using a rolling pin.

5. Spray the pressure cooker with the olive oil inside and transfer the rolled dough there.

6. Add the salmon mixture and flatten it well. Wrap the edges of the dough and close the lid.

7. Cook the pie for 35 minutes on the "Pressure" mode. When the pie is done, let it cool briefly.

8. Remove it from the pressure cooker and slice it. Serve it warm.

Nutrition: calories 515, fat 44.3, fiber 3.6, carbs 11.7, protein 16.8

Onion French Soup

Prep time: 15 minutes

Cooking time: 25 minutes

Servings: 6

Ingredients:

- 1 pound yellow onions
- 1 cup cream
- 4 cups beef stock
- 1 teaspoon salt
- 1 teaspoon ground black pepper
- 1 teaspoon turmeric
- ½ teaspoon nutmeg
- 1 teaspoon cilantro
- ½ teaspoon white pepper
- 1 medium carrot
- 2 ounces unsalted butter

Directions:

1. Peel the onions and carrot. Dice the onion and grate the carrot.

2. Combine the vegetables together and sprinkle the mixture with the salt, ground black pepper, turmeric, nutmeg, cilantro, and white pepper.

3. Blend the mixture.

4. Add the unsalted butter in the pressure cooker and melt it. Add the onion mixture and sauté the vegetables until they are golden brown, stirring frequently.

5. Add beef stock and cream. Stir the mixture well and set the pressure cooker mode to "Sauté." Close the lid and cook the soup for 15 minutes.

6. When the cooking time ends, remove the soup from the pressure cooker and let it cool briefly.

7. Ladle it into the serving bowls and serve it.

Nutrition: calories 277, fat 23.8, fiber 2, carbs 11.58, protein 5

Gnocchi

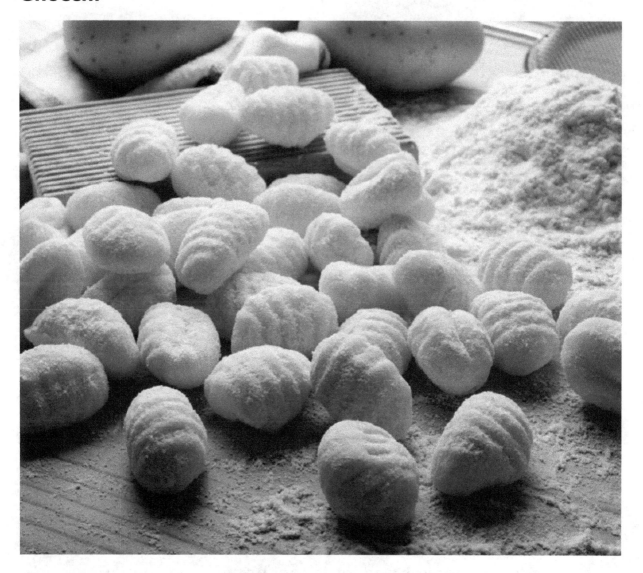

Prep time: 10 minutes

Cooking time: 15 minutes

Servings: 4

Ingredients:

- 8 ounces turnip, flaked
- ½ cup coconut flour
- 1 teaspoon salt
- 4 cups of water
- 1 teaspoon oregano
- ½ teaspoon white pepper
- 1 teaspoon paprika

Directions:

1. Transfer the turnip in the pressure cooker.
2. Add coconut flour, 1 cup of water, salt, oregano, paprika, and white pepper.
3. Stir the mixture gently and close the lid.
4. Set the manual mode and cook for 10 minutes.
5. Blend well and remove it from the pressure cooker.
6. Knead the dough and separate it into the small balls, or gnocchi. Pour 3 cups of the water in the pressure cooker and preheat it.

7. Transfer the gnocchi to the preheated water and stir the mixture well. Close the lid, and set the pressure cooker mode to "Steam."

8. Cook for 7 to 10 minutes or until they are cooked.

9. Remove the dish from the pressure cooker and transfer to the serving plate. Chill it briefly and add your favorite sauce.

Nutrition: calories 89, fat 2.7, fiber 7.5, carbs 13.4, protein 3.7

Mozzarella Pie

Prep time: 15 minutes

Cooking time: 30 minutes

Servings: 8

Ingredients:

- 1 pound rutabaga
- 8 ounces sliced bacon
- 1 onion
- ½ cup cream
- 1 tablespoon olive oil
- 1 teaspoon salt
- 1 teaspoon cilantro
- 1 teaspoon oregano
- ½ teaspoon red chili pepper
- 5 ounces Mozzarella cheese

Directions:

1. Slice the bacon and sprinkle it with the salt and cilantro and stir the mixture.

2. Peel the rutabaga and slice it. Spray the pressure cooker with the olive oil inside. Add half of the sliced bacon into the pressure cooker.

3. Add the sliced rutabaga and sprinkle it with the oregano and red chili pepper. Peel the onion and slice it. Slice the Mozzarella cheese.

4. Add the sliced ingredients in the pressure cooker pie. Pour the cream.

5. Cover the pie with the second half of the sliced bacon and close the lid. Set the pressure cooker mode to "Pressure," and cook for 30 minutes.

6. Release the pressure and check if the pie is cooked.

7. Remove the pie from the pressure cooker and chill it well. Cut the cooked dish into pieces and serve.

Nutrition: calories 255, fat 17.7, fiber 1.8, carbs 7.6, protein 16.5

Herbed Chicken Wings

Prep time: 15 minutes

Cooking time: 10 minutes

Servings: 6

Ingredients:

- 12 chicken wings, bones removed
- 1 tablespoon oregano
- 1 teaspoon paprika
- 1 teaspoon turmeric
- ½ teaspoon salt
- 2 tablespoons butter, melted
- 1 teaspoon cayenne pepper
- ½ teaspoon olive oil
- ½ teaspoon minced garlic

Directions:

1. Make the chicken marinade: mix up together oregano, paprika, turmeric, salt, melted butter, cayenne pepper, olive oil, and minced garlic.
2. Whisk the mixture well. Then brush every chicken wing with marinade and leave for 10 minutes to marinate.
3. After this, transfer the chicken wings into the cooker basket and lower the crisp lid.
4. Cook the chicken wings for 10 minutes or until they are light brown.

Nutrition: calories 361, fat 25.8, fiber 0.9, carbs 11.9, protein 19.7

Halloumi Salad with Beef Tenderloins

Prep time: 15 minutes

Cooking time: 10 minutes

Servings: 6

Ingredients:

- 7 ounces halloumi cheese
- 1 tablespoon orange juice
- 1 teaspoon sesame oil
- ½ teaspoon cumin
- ½ cup arugula
- 1 pound beef tenderloins
- 1 tablespoon lemon juice
- 1 teaspoon apple cider vinegar
- 1 teaspoon salt
- 1 teaspoon ground white pepper
- 1 tablespoon olive oil
- 1 teaspoon rosemary
- 1 cup romaine lettuce

Directions:

1. Tenderize the beef tenderloins well and cover them with the cumin, lemon juice, apple cider vinegar, ground white pepper, salt, and rosemary.

2. Marinate the meat for at least 10 minutes.

3. Transfer the meat to the pressure cooker and sauté for 10 minutes or until it is cooked. Flip it into another side from time to time.

4. Chop the beef tenderloins roughly and transfer them to the serving bowl. Tear the lettuce and add it to the meat bowl.

5. Slice the halloumi cheese and sprinkle it with the sesame oil.

6. Chop the arugula. Add the ingredients to the meat mixture.

7. Sprinkle the salad with the orange juice and mix well. Serve the salad immediately.

Nutrition: calories 289, fat 16.9, fiber 0, carbs 4.53, protein 29

Basil Pho

Prep time: 15 minutes

Cooking time: 32 minutes

Servings: 9

Ingredients:

- 5 cups of water
- 4 ounces scallions
- 3 ounces shallot
- 1 teaspoon salt
- 1 teaspoon paprika
- ½ tablespoon red chili flakes
- 1 teaspoon ground white pepper
- ⅓ cup fresh basil
- 1 tablespoon garlic sauce
- 2 medium onions
- ½ lime
- 1 teaspoon nutmeg
- 2 pounds of chicken breast

Directions:

1. Peel the onions and slice them. Place the sliced onions in the pressure cooker.

2. Chop the shallot and scallions and add them in the pressure cooker too.

3. Sprinkle the mixture with the ground white pepper, chili flakes, paprika, salt, and nutmeg. Stir the mixture and sauté it for 30 seconds.

4. Add water and the chicken breast. Close the lid and cook the mixture at the pressure mode for 30 minutes.

5. When the cooking time ends, release the remaining pressure and remove the chicken from the water.

6. Strain the water using a colander. Shred the chicken.

7. Add the shredded chicken in the serving bowls.

8. Sprinkle the dish with the garlic sauce. Squeeze lime juice from the lime and add the liquid to the dish. Stir it gently and serve immediately.

Nutrition: calories 139, fat 2.7, fiber 1.2, carbs 5.6, protein 22.2

Butter Asparagus Pie

Prep time: 15 minutes

Cooking time: 30 minutes

Servings: 8

Ingredients:

- 10 ounces butter
- 3 cups almond flour
- 1 egg
- 1 teaspoon salt
- 1 pound asparagus
- 2 tablespoons olive oil
- ½ cup pork rind
- 1 teaspoon paprika
- ½ cup dill

Directions:

1. Combine the soft butter, almond flour, and egg together in a mixing bowl. Knead the dough until smooth.

2. Chop the asparagus and dill. Combine the chopped vegetables together.

3. Sprinkle the mixture with the salt, half of the pork rinds, and paprika. Blend the mixture. Transfer the dough to the pressure cooker and flatten it well.

4. Add the chopped asparagus mixture. Sprinkle the pie with the pork rinds.

5. Sprinkle the pie with the olive oil and close the lid. Cook the pie at the pressure mode for 30 minutes.

6. When the dish is cooked, release the remaining pressure and let the pie rest. Cut it into pieces and serve.

Nutrition: calories 622, fat 58, fiber 6.2, carbs 11.6, protein 7.4

Enoki Mushroom Soup

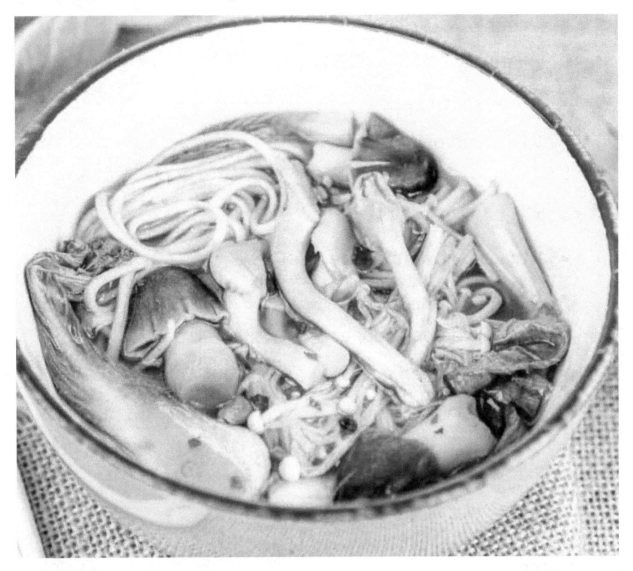

Prep time: 15 minutes

Cooking time: 50 minutes

Servings: 8

Ingredients:

- 1 cup Enoki mushrooms
- 7 cups of water
- 1 cup dill
- 4 tablespoons salsa
- 1 jalapeno pepper
- ⅓ cup cream
- 2 teaspoons salt
- 1 teaspoon white pepper
- 1 white onion
- 1 sweet red bell pepper
- 1 pound chicken breast
- 1 teaspoon soy sauce

Directions:

1. Place Enoki mushrooms in the pressure cooker.

2. Chop the chicken breast and add it in the pressure cooker. Add water and cook the mushrooms at the pressure mode for 35 minutes.

3. Meanwhile, chop the dill and jalapeno peppers. Slice the onions and chop the bell pepper.

4. Add the vegetables to bean mixture and close the lid. Set the pressure cooker mode to "Pressure," and cook for 15 minutes.

5. Sprinkle the soup with the cream, salsa, white pepper, and soy sauce.

6. Stir the soup and cook it for 5 minutes.

7. Remove the soup from the pressure cooker and let it rest briefly. Ladle the soup into the serving bowls.

Nutrition: calories 101, fat 2.3, fiber 1.6, carbs 6.7, protein 13.9

Conclusion

Being an excellent service both for immediate pot beginners and knowledgeable instant pot users this immediate pot cookbook boosts your day-to-day food preparation. It makes you look like a professional and cook like a pro. Thanks to the Immediate Pot component, this cookbook assists you with preparing straightforward and tasty meals for any budget. Satisfy everybody with hearty suppers, nutritious breakfasts, sweetest desserts, as well as enjoyable treats. Despite if you cook for one or prepare bigger sections-- there's a service for any type of feasible cooking circumstance. Boost your methods on how to cook in one of the most effective means making use of just your split second pot, this recipe book, and some perseverance to find out quick. Valuable ideas and also methods are discreetly incorporated into every recipe to make your household request new meals time and time again. Vegan options, solutions for meat-eaters and extremely satisfying ideas to unify the entire household at the same table. Consuming in your home is a common experience, as well as it can be so great to fulfill completely at the end of the day. Master your Instant Pot as well as take advantage of this brand-new experience beginning today!